Table of Contents

The F-Factor Diet

The F-Factor Diet is a popular weight loss program that has helped many people achieve their weight loss goals. The diet focuses on increasing your intake of fiber and lean proteins while reducing your consumption of unhealthy foods.

The first step of the F-Factor Diet is to cut out unhealthy foods such as refined carbohydrates, processed foods, and added sugars. You should also reduce your consumption of saturated fats and replace them with healthier monounsaturated and polyunsaturated fats.

The second step of the F-Factor Diet is to increase your intake of high-fiber foods such as vegetables, fruits, and whole grains. Eating a high-fiber diet can help keep you feeling full and can also reduce your risk of developing certain diseases.

The third step of the F-Factor Diet is to increase your intake of lean proteins such as lean meats, fish, eggs, and beans. Eating a diet high in lean proteins can help to build and maintain muscle mass and can also help to keep you feeling full.

The fourth step of the F-Factor Diet is to create a caloric deficit. This means that you should be eating fewer calories than you are burning. This can be done by cutting out unhealthy foods and replacing them with healthier options.

By following the F-Factor Diet, you can easily achieve your weight loss goals. Just remember to keep your goals realistic and to reward yourself along the way. With dedication and perseverance, you will be able to reach your ultimate weight loss goals.

Sarah's Story

When Sarah first heard about the F-Factor Diet, she was skeptical. She had tried countless diets in the past, but none of them had worked. But the F-Factor Diet promised something different - a way to lose weight without giving up the foods she loved. So she decided to give it a try.

After a few weeks, Sarah noticed that she was beginning to lose weight. She found that the F-Factor Diet was easy to stick to and that she wasn't feeling as hungry as she used to. She was also able to eat some of her favorite foods, like pizza and ice cream, without feeling guilty.

As the weeks passed, Sarah's weight loss continued and she felt more energized than ever before. She was able to stay active and even started to enjoy exercising.

After several months of following the F-Factor Diet, Sarah had lost an incredible thirty pounds. She was amazed by her results and felt healthier and happier than ever before.

The F-Factor Diet worked for Sarah, and it can work for you too. With its focus on fiber, lean protein, and healthy fats, the F-Factor Diet can help you lose weight and feel your best. So why not give it a try?

All that You Need to Know About the F-Factor Diet

With regards to smart dieting, we're about a decent methodology that fills our plate with scrumptious and fulfilling nourishments to keep us stimulated throughout the day. And keeping in mind that most prevailing fashion eats less carbs have their second at that point blur away, The F-Factor Diet is one that has stood the trial of time, and in light of current circumstances. Its methodology centers around joining protein and fiber, the thought being that this specific combo keeps you feeling full for the duration of the day, taking out the hardship that a great many people understanding on conventional "consumes less calories." It's no big surprise that celebs like Katie Couric, Megyn Kelley, and even Miss Universe depend on the arrangement, likely in light of the fact that it doesn't expect you to boycott starches, proteins, fats, or even liquor. Which means: you can really have a public activity without tumbling off the cart.

With F-Factor, the truth will eventually come out – it's a healthfully solid way to deal with eating forever that really gives you more decisions for what to eat while attempting to get more fit, not less.

At its center, F-Factor is established in a fundamental logical comprehension of life systems and physiology that its organizer, Tanya Zuckerbrot read for more than 20 years in her profession as a Registered Dietitian. Since F-

Factor has as of late experienced a resurgence (we've genuinely been finding out about it wherever of late) our interest drove us directly to the lady herself, who thoughtfully gave us the full scoop.

How Did F-Factor come to fruition?

The F-Factor Diet was a result of my initial work as a Registered Dietitian, when I went about as an expansion of the clinical group of clinical patients with conditions like cardiovascular sickness and diabetes. At the time my activity was to make feast designs that would bring down the cholesterol of cardiovascular patients or, on account of the diabetics, help to deal with their glucose levels. Both patient populaces got forms of a high fiber abstains from food as a result of fiber's capacity to bring down cholesterol and oversee glucose levels. The patients got more beneficial – cholesterol improved, sugars were better overseen, and suddenly, in all cases, these patients shed pounds. The customers were carrying on with their lives typically, appreciating suppers at their preferred cafés, drinking liquor, and getting more beneficial all the while.

What I had not foreseen was that by recommending such a great amount of fiber for the clinical advantages, these patients were just inclination more full for the duration of the day on less calories, which prompted weight reduction without hunger. Companions and partners of theirs saw as well and brought in, mentioning counts calories for themselves, yet for the weight reduction benefits simply, not to deal with their sugars or cholesterol. This was the introduction of the F-Factor Diet and the training kept on developing from that point.

How It Works

This is unmistakably not simply one more 'prevailing fashion diet'. How can it work to deliver such astounding outcomes, without a gigantic change in way of life?

The F-Factor Diet is a maintainable way to deal with changeless weight reduction and ideal wellbeing. The overall ideas driving the program clarify why it can such stunning outcomes (individuals can hope to lose up to 15 lbs. in the principal month!), without an enormous way of life change.

Where most eating regimens depend on hardship, (advising you to remove certain nourishments), F-Factor is about what nourishments to include into your eating routine so as to get thinner. This makes F-Factor both economical and freeing, which is the reason individuals succeed and remain on it longterm. F-Factor works on account of fiber — the mystery supplement for getting in shape without hunger. Fiber is the zero-calorie, non-edible piece of a starch that adds mass to food.

Fiber, explicitly, is basic to progress on the F-Factor Diet, as it permits you to eat the starches vital for vitality without putting on weight. It swells in the stomach, retains and evacuates fat and calories, and lifts digestion. At the point when you follow an eating routine wealthy in fiber you feel full in the wake of eating – so you'll by and large eat less for the duration of the day.

Likewise, fiber is constantly matched with protein. Clinical proof shows that fiber and protein have a high satiety advantage in calorie-controlled eating regimens and in weight decrease. The mix of fiber and protein keeps you feeling full, for the longest timeframe, on the least calories. The more full you feel after a dinner, the more outlandish you'll be to gorge at the following supper; and, along these lines, the almost certain you'll be to get more fit.

Fiber and protein at each feast makes getting thinner no biggie!

On F-Factor, you eat 4 dinners for each day and follow this example at every feast. F-Factor calorie counters are empowered/intend to eat 4 suppers every day – breakfast, lunch, bite, and supper, at 4-5 hour spans. What the vast majority don't know is that when your body is denied of nourishment for a long time between dinners, it begins preserving fuel and consuming less calories to shield itself from starving. Your digestion eases back down, accordingly restraining weight reduction in spite of decreased caloric admission. Additionally, glucose levels start to drop inside two hours of eating. Low glucose can create abrupt food cravings, which can trigger gorging and food desires. Following the F-Factor design with high fiber nourishments makes it simple to shed pounds without hunger.

The Eating Plan

What are some key parts of the eating plan?

F-Factor works on the grounds that not at all like different eating regimens, you're not ravenous for the duration of the day, and it's practical. F-Factor depends on 4 problematic rules that are outlandish to all that we accept about the weight reduction space:

Eat carbs. The privilege carbs are filling, low in calories and lift digestion

Feast out. On F-Factor you can eat out from Day 1 as no menu is forbidden!

Drink liquor. Consuming less calories and social drinking can go all together, solid way of life.

Exercise less. On F-Factor you'll shed pounds and fabricate slender muscle without going through hours at the rec center.

Along these lines, while the F in F-Factor represents fiber, which makes for weight reduction without hunger, it likewise represents opportunity.

On F-Factor, you have the opportunity to feast out anyplace, or cook for yourself in the event that you need. You have the opportunity to drink liquor and all the more spare time as well, since existence with F-Factor doesn't expect you to go through hours at the rec center.

Why F-Factor Is Different

What sets F-Factor separated from different weight control plans?

The larger key territories where F-Factor is unique in relation to different weight control plans are:

Oversight versus expansion: Most eating regimens depend on exclusion—to achieve weight reduction, certain nourishments like starches or fats, or lifestyles, such as feasting out or drinking, are discarded. The issue with this is it leaves weight watchers feeling denied and disappointed.

F-Factor depends on option—you add fiber into your eating regimen to get thinner, so there are no sentiments of yearning and disavowal, which regularly makes weight watchers come up short.

It's freeing: F-Factor is intended to fit flawlessly into people groups' lives so they can stay on course, and the arrangement turns into their new typical.

At its center, F-Factor is about training. It shows individuals how to eat forever, and how to keep up their weight reduction (which amends the major issue of prevailing fashion abstains from food). With most weight reduction plans, weight reduction eases back and turns out to be more troublesome as the weight falls off, on the grounds that digestion eases back. On F-Factor, the weight reduction proceeds and doesn't level in light of the fact that the fiber keeps on firing up the digestion. Individuals on other eating routine plans will in general get disheartened and surrender when their advancement eases back, on F-Factor there is no compelling reason to feel debilitated, which likewise adds to it being a feasible lifestyle.

Three Periods Of The F-Factor Diet

Depict the periods of the F-Factor plan? What is permitted on the dinner plan for each stage?

There are three periods of The F-Factor Diet—kick off your weight reduction, proceeded with weight reduction, and upkeep—We call these Step 1, Step 2 and Step 3. As you progress from Step 1 to Step 2 to Step 3 you are including extra servings of sugars every day to your eating regimen.

Stage 1: Jump Start Your Weight Loss

The reason for Step 1 is to help weight reduction quickly – the main starches permitted are a high-fiber grain, high-fiber GG saltines, a serving of natural product, F-Factor 20/20 Fiber/Protein powder, and F-Factor bars. Stage 1 of the eating routine is intended to support weight reduction and help slide you into the eating regimen. It necessitates that you cut out specific nourishments for just fourteen days.

Stage 1 Guidelines:

3 servings of starches/day — (1 serving of sugars = 15g of carbs).

Focus on 35 grams of fiber and under 35 grams of net sugars every day.

During this stage starches and bland vegetables, more than one serving of natural product, most dairy, and medium-to high-fat meats are to be stayed away from.

In the wake of being on Step 1 for about fourteen days, you graduate to Step 2 and add three servings of sugars to your stage 1 eating plan.

Stage 2: Continued Weight Loss

Stage 2 copies Step 1 generally; be that as it may, this area of the eating routine calls for three additional servings of sugars a day. The decision of the sugar is up to you. You can include more organic product, pasta, a bagel, and so forth. – it's everything up to you. These decisions make this eating routine so inconceivably simple and reasonable. You can change what you eat while following the arrangement. In the wake of completing Step 2, you presently know which nourishments are fiber-overwhelming and how to explore a solid eating regimen.

Stage 2 Guidelines:

6 servings of sugars/day — (1 serving of starches = 15g of carbs).

Focus on in any event 35 grams of fiber and under 75 grams of net sugars every day.

Since you can have 3 extra servings of sugars here you can include starches and bland vegetables in.

Adhere to a Step 2 eating plan until you arrive at your objective load before moving onto Step 3.

Stage 3: Maintenance-Eating forever

Stage 3 means three additional servings of starches to what you have been doing in Step 2. When that you arrive at Step 3, you realize how to explore eating in an eatery or a market, and how to set up your own food.

Stage 3 Guidelines:

9 servings of sugars/day–(1 serving of starches = 15g of carbs).

Focus on in any event 35 grams of fiber and under 125 grams of net sugars every day.

Stage 3 is much the same as Step 2, yet include three additional servings of sugars.

Keep in mind, you can generally return to Steps 1 and 2 in the event that you need to lose more

What changes do individuals will in general notification with each stage?

Individuals see and feel results after as meager as multi week of following the program. Not exclusively does weight reduction happen in the absolute first week, numerous customers report improved rest and vitality, laxation, and feel engaged to stay on track.

The normal weight reduction following one month on the program is 8-10 pounds for ladies, and 15-20 pounds for men.

Whenever followed precisely (no cheating), one can hope to lose 4-6 lbs in the initial fourteen days on Step 1. Notwithstanding weight reduction, you can hope to have improved your digestion, experienced less emotional episodes and sentiments of weariness, rested better, felt less enlarged, and had less yearnings for sugars. At the point when you include more starches in the two Steps 2 and 3, you will see an expansion in your vitality levels just as extra weight reduction.

Fiber = Your BFF

Clarify the superpowers of fiber and advantages one can procure by including more fiber into their eating routine?

Fiber adds mass to food without including calories, which is the reason high-fiber nourishments are incredible for eating fewer carbs. It likewise grows in the stomach, eases back absorption, and lifts digestion, and this consolidated to make shedding pounds more advantageous and simpler. What truly gives fiber its wonder status is the manner in which it absorbs and expels fat and calories in the stomach before your body can retain them. Staggeringly, the fiber found in tasty, nutritious, filling carbs does what no other food can – it really causes fat and calories to vanish!

Fiber is the zero-calorie, non-absorbable piece of a sugar that adds mass to food. It has significant wellbeing and health benefits, and is key for weight reduction and the executives.

Different advantages of eating a fiber-rich eating routine

Expanded vitality: Eating fiber and protein together keeps blood glucose levels consistent, giving your body continued vitality.

Compliment stomach: Eating a high-fiber diet causes you have total and normal solid discharges. Fiber builds stool mass, which forestalls obstruction, swelling and can offer alleviation from bad tempered inside condition.

More clear skin: Fiber absorbs poisons in the blood and kills them through the stomach related lot rather than your pores, delivering more splendid, more clear skin. Numerous fiber-rich foods grown from the ground are wealthy in cancer prevention agents that help battle maturing.

Improved rest: Eating refined carbs late in the day cause your glucose level to top and afterward crash during rest, which is the reason a few people get up in the center of the night. Eating nourishments wealthy in fiber assists keep with blooding sugars consistent, which thusly advances undisturbed rest.

Most loved fiber-rich nourishments?

Fiber is found in a wide range of nourishments. Most loved fiber-rich nourishments include:

F-Factor 20/20 Fiber/Protein Powder: It is a lot higher in fiber than other protein powders (most whey protein powders have 1-2g fiber per serving, vegetable protein powders have ~9g, and this powder has 20g)

Natural products: bananas, oranges, apples, mangoes, strawberries, raspberries.

Vegetables: for the most part, the more obscure the shading, the higher the fiber content. Top off your shopping basket with: carrots, beets, broccoli, collard greens, swiss chard, spinach, artichokes, potatoes (chestnut, red, and sweet).

Beans and Legumes: Beans and vegetables are tasty, fiber-filled increments to plates of mixed greens, soups, and stews. Naval force, white, garbanzo, kidney, peas, or lentils are on the whole sound decisions.

Breads and Grains: GG Crackers, entire addition breads, Wheat Bran or other high fiber oats.

Cooking With F-Factor

I am so glad for my items! My F-Factor 20/20 Fiber/Protein Powder is actually a saint element for anybody hoping to deal with their weight or improve their wellbeing. It is totally not normal for whatever else accessible today – the powder has multiple times more fiber than some other protein powder accessible to date. The "20/20" alludes to the measure of fiber and protein in a serving—one serving (2 scoops) packs 20 grams of fat-battling fiber to help digestion, alongside 20 grams of natural muscle-building protein, for only 150 calories. The powder is additionally sans gluten, without soy, has no sugar included, and is all characteristic, non-GMO, and Kosher.

While it was initially planned for use in smoothies and shakes, it has immediately become a staple fixing in individuals' kitchens. It comes in both a chocolate and vanilla flavor, and can be utilized to upgrade the supplement thickness of incalculable dishes; everything from waffles to flapjacks, cakes and treats, frozen yogurt, and biscuits. I like to add them to espresso to make a scrumptious fiber-filled latte, or use them in plans like waffles and biscuits to fulfill that sweet tooth.

What are your most loved go-to weeknight plans?

A portion of my preferred family supper plans are remembered for the new form of the F-Factor Diet Book, as zoodles with mozzarella-stuffed meatballs (YUM!). I likewise love making F-Factor Chili with a DIY fixings bar, and my go-to taco night. We add new plans to our site consistently, as well!

A portion of my top choices include:

- Eggplant Parmesan Lasagna
- Waffles and Muffins made with 20/20 Fiber/Protein powder

- 10 Vegetable Soup

- Guiltless Chicken Parmesan

- Asian Sesame Snap Pea Salad

- Bar-b-que Chicken Cauliflower Crust Pizza

Enlisted dietitian Tanya Zuckerbrot considers fiber the "supernatural occurrence carb." She cherishes it such a great amount, actually, she structured a whole eating regimen around it. Since 2007, fans have been following her book of scriptures The F-Factor Diet, and Zuckerbrot claims the normal F-

Factor health food nut sheds 8 to 10 pounds in the main month—without yearning or sentiments of hardship. What's more, it's making waves again after another examination survey distributed in The Lancet found that the individuals who eat more fiber (between 25 to 29 grams for each day) diminish their danger of kicking the bucket from cardiovascular ailment by 15 to 30 percent, contrasted with the individuals who eat around 20 grams or less every day. (See: This Study On Carbs Might Make You Rethink Your Keto Diet Aspirations)

So is Zuckerbrot loaded with it—or has she at long last discovered a weight reduction answer for the individuals who would prefer not to include calories or kick it in ketosis on the keto diet?

What Is the F-Factor Diet, Exactly?

"The F-Factor Diet is a way of life that centers around expending high-fiber sugars joined with protein at each feast to keep you fulfilled and permit you to get thinner while devouring less calories," clarifies Lauren Harris-Pincus, M.S., R.D.N., organizer of NutritionStarringYOU.com and creator of The Protein-Packed Breakfast Club. "In addition, beside weight reduction, the medical advantages of fiber, for example, improved cholesterol, glucose, consistency, and supported vitality levels are a side reward."

Around 95 percent of Americans don't verge on hitting the measure of every day fiber suggested by the U.S. Dietary Guidelines, says Harris-Pincus, which is 14 grams for each 1,000 calories or around 25 grams for ladies and 38 grams for men every day. The F-Factor advances focusing on at least 35 grams every day and following them by means of a food diary to keep yourself responsible. Zuckerbrot even offers a model diary and extra tips on her site, and she suggests three suppers and one nibble for each day.

There's zero advancement of activity on the F-Factor diet. Truth be told, Zuckerbrot proposes evading cardio, specifically, saying that it expands your hunger so much that you'll wind up eating a greater number of calories than you consume.

What Can You Eat On the F-Factor Diet?

The F-Factor diet centers around "net carbs".

Since carbs from fiber aren't absorbable, "you deduct the fiber content from the all out sugar on the mark to show up at 'net carbs', which means the grams of carbs that are accessible for absorption by the body," says Harris-Pincus. (BTW, here's actually what number of carbs you ought to eat a day.)

F-Factor calorie counters follow a few stages and increment all out net carb utilization as they inch nearer to their objective.

Stage 1: Less than 35 grams net carbs every day, or around three servings

Stage 2: Less than 75 grams net carbs every day, or around six servings

Upkeep Phase: Less than 125 grams net carbs every day, or around nine servings

Low-net carb nourishments Zuckerbrot suggests while on the F-Factor diet:

Beans and vegetables all things considered

Eggs

High-fiber vegetables, for example, beets, broccoli, carrots, cauliflower, and yams

High-fiber natural products including apples, berries, oranges, and pears

Nut spread

GG Crackers

High-fiber grains

Entire wheat bread (P.S. Here's the distinction between entire wheat and entire grain.) She likewise sells F-Factor protein powder and bars for extra in a hurry choices. Liquor (wine, spirits with without calorie blenders) is allowed, as long as utilization is with some restraint and inside your every day net carb limits. (Related: Your Guide to Drinking Alcohol On the Keto Diet)

"It's shockingly simple to follow when feasting out and going with a couple of straightforward replacements," says Harris-Pincus.

What Is The F-Factor Diet

Tanya Zuckerbrot, the originator of the F-Factor Diet is the genius behind this good dieting arrangement. Zuckerbrot has more than 20 years of experience as a Registered Dietitian yet it was in the previous long stretches of her profession that she made the revelation of this astonishing eating routine. Zuckerbrot worked with a clinical group to make an extraordinary high-fiber supper plan in would like to help individuals with conditions like cardiovascular infection and diabetes. Every patient was given an adaptation of a high-fiber diet since fiber can help lower cholesterol and oversee glucose levels.

Not exclusively was the eating plan helping the patients, yet they additionally announced that they felt all the more full, for more, which caused them to devour less calories and at long last, likewise brought about weight reduction. This was a symptom Zuckerbrot didn't foresee and is basically how the eating routine bloomed. From that point on companions and associates started mentioning the eating regimen plan and now numerous individuals around the globe are evaluating this eating regimen for themselves.

Why The F-Factor Diet Works

Fortunately with the F-Factor Diet, you don't need to deny yourself of specific nourishments to get more fit and this is a central motivation behind why it's so reasonable. This eating routine urges you to enjoy high-fiber, protein-rich nourishments that will assist you with feeling all the more full for more. All things considered, you're additionally still urged to appreciate carbs, fats, and even liquor. So fortunately with this eating regimen, you can at present have a public activity!

The F-Factor diet puts a major accentuation on a not all that mystery supplement — fiber! For those that don't have a clue, fiber is the zero-calorie, non-edible piece of starches. An eating routine wealthy in fiber will assist you with feeling all the more full in the wake of eating and will urge you to eat less for the duration of the day.

The Benefits Of Fiber

Fiber has numerous different advantages beside weight reduction. At the point when fiber is joined with protein, blood glucose levels will avoid spiking and dropping radically which will bring about expanded vitality and may even improve your rest. Fiber likewise adds mass to your stool which will help advance customary solid discharges and forestall obstruction and swelling.

Further, fiber can likewise assimilate poisons in the blood and afterward discard them through the stomach related parcel rather than through our pores which can result in more clear skin. Foods grown from the ground likewise contain cancer prevention agents which advance more clear skin as well as battle maturing as well.

How The F-Factor Diet Works

While following this supper plan you'll enjoy 4 suppers for every day; breakfast, lunch, tidbit, and supper. It's critical to eat each 4 to 5 hours in such a case that you deny your assortment of nourishment for a really long time, it will begin to preserve fuel by consuming less calories and may even lull your digestion. Further, in the event that you permit your glucose to drop excessively low, you may encounter exceptional food longings and for a few, it can trigger pigging out.

The eating regimen works in 3 stages; stage 1, stage 2 and stage 3. Stage 1 spotlights on kicking off your weight reduction while stage 2 spotlights on proceeded with weight reduction. At long last, stage 3 puts a major accentuation on upkeep so you can stay aware of these smart dieting propensities without tumbling off the cart. We should plunge into this more next.

Stage 1: Jump-Starting Your Weight Loss

Stage 1 is somewhat prohibitive however this is simply because the objective is to support your digestion and start weight reduction right away. It's likewise significant that you'll just be limiting sure nourishments for about fourteen days. In this stage, you should cut all carbs aside from high-fiber grains, high fiber GG Crackers (we'll talk more about these later), F-Factor protein powder, F-Factor bars, and a serving of natural product.

It's critical to have 2 servings of carbs every day with each serving being 15 grams of carbs. Make certain to focus on 35 grams of fiber and under 35 grams of net carbs (to figure, take away fiber and sugar liquor from the aggregate sum of carbs) every day. You'll likewise need to maintain a strategic distance from starches, bland vegetables, more than one serving of organic product, most dairy, and medium to high-fat meats.

Stage 2: Continued Weight Loss

Stage 2 is very like stage 1, however this time you're ready to include 3 additional servings of carbs every day. This time you get the chance to pick your carbs whether it be pasta, a bagel, more natural product, or whatever your heart wants (sensibly speaking, obviously).

In this stage, you'll despite everything need to focus on 35 grams of fiber for every day, nonetheless, since the carbs have expanded, you would now be able to expend under 75 grams of net carbs every day. You're likewise now ready to begin including starches including dull vegetables. During this stage, you should start to have an away from of which nourishments are wealthy in fiber.

Stage 3: Maintenance

Since you've started up your digestion it's an ideal opportunity to begin the support stage. In this stage, you can indicate an extra 3 additional servings of carbs. By and by, focus on 35 grams of fiber for each day however now you can expend under 125 grams of net carbs every day.

When you progress into the upkeep stage you should start to feel more good shopping at the market, setting up your own food just as exploring a menu at an eatery. In the event that you might want to lose more weight you can basically enter stages 1 or 2 again and afterward advance back to the support stage once you've arrived at your ideal weight.

What Can You Expect From The F-Factor Diet

When you leave on this good dieting venture, there are many positive reactions you can anticipate. First off, those that can follow the arrangement precisely how it is — with no cheating — ought to have the option to lose around 4 to 6 pounds in the initial fourteen days and up to 8 to 10 pounds in the principal month.

In any case, beside weight reduction, you can likewise hope to feel less swelling, experience more vitality and less weakness, your rest may improve, you may encounter less emotional episodes, and you may likewise encounter less yearnings for carbs. Next, how about we plunge into some flavorful fiber-rich nourishments you can eat now.

High-Fiber Fruits

There are numerous high fiber natural products that would make an incredible expansion to your day by day diet. Also, organic products are normally sweet making it the ideal food to extinguish a sweet tooth wanting. On your next staple outing make certain to get bananas, oranges, strawberries, and apples as these natural products contain around 3 to 4 grams of fiber for each serving. When eating apples make certain to eat the strip as it contains the most sum fiber.

Other magnificent choices incorporate raspberries which contain around 8 grams of fiber for each cup and extraordinary organic products, for example, mangos, persimmon, and guava which contain around 5 to 9 grams of fiber for every serving.

High-Fiber Vegetables

An overall principle you'll need to remember when loading up on high fiber veggies is 'the more obscure the shading, the higher the fiber'. Some extraordinary high-fiber vegetables are carrots, beets, collard greens, broccoli, swiss chard, spinach, artichokes, and potatoes.

It's important that artichokes are one of the most fiber-rich veggies as they contain around 10 grams of fiber in one medium-sized artichoke. Further, when buying potatoes, search for reddish brown, red, or yams and make certain to eat the skin. Much the same as apples, this is the place you can discover a large portion of the fiber content.

High-Fiber Grains

Entire grains are an incredible expansion to numerous suppers that will keep you feeling full for more. Some incredible high-fiber grains incorporate entire grain bread, Wheat Bran, and other high fiber oats.

GG Crackers are additionally profoundly energized on this eating regimen. They can be utilized as a substitute to bread, as a fixing to serving of mixed greens, sprinkled on head of macintosh and cheddar and that's only the tip of the iceberg! Need to attempt them?

High-Fiber Beans/Legumes

Beans and vegetables make an incredible expansion to soups, stews, and plates of mixed greens. Some extraordinary high-fiber choices incorporate naval force, white, garbanzo (chickpeas), kidney beans, peas, and lentils.

Need to attempt a fiber-rich feast that is brimming with generous flavorful beans? Attempt this F-

Factor Homestyle Chili formula HERE. In addition to the fact that it is loaded with fiber it's flooding in delectable flavor as well.

F-Factor Products

There are a few F-Factor items accessible to assist you with remaining on target. To start, F-Factor has 3 protein powders to look over — chocolate, vanilla, and unflavored. Every protein powder gives 20 grams of protein and 20 grams of fiber for every serving. The unflavored powder is an extraordinary alternative to add to prepared dinners and heated merchandise to help that fiber content easily.

Further F-Factor additionally has an incredible determination of protein bars to browse including blueberry, chocolate brownie, and nutty spread. These bars make in a hurry snacks simple and available.

Tips For Success On The F-Factor Diet

Following an eating routine requires inspiration and commitment however there are some different tips and apparatuses that can assist you with being fruitful as well. First off, you might need to have a go at journaling so you can follow the nourishments you eat (to guarantee you're expending enough fiber), your feelings, rest designs, and your weight. Along these lines you'll have the option to effectively think back and ponder your advance and decide territories you can enhance.

You could likewise consider finding a responsibility accomplice whether that be your accomplice, a relative, or a companion. Having an emotionally supportive network as you change into this sound way of life will just urge you to continue onward. At last, you can likewise remain associated with the F-Factor Instagram account where they share tips and plans each day. Be that as it may, the vast majority of all, ensure you mess around with it! Next, we should take a gander at some heavenly high-fiber plans you can begin getting a charge out of now!

Need to remain on target? Look at this feast organizer diary.

Breakfast: Waffles

Jump into a scrumptious plate of cushioned hotcakes with this F-Factor-affirmed formula! These waffles are high in fiber as well as they're sans gluten as well.

On the off chance that you don't have a waffle producer don't worry, the hitter can be utilized to make heavenly flapjacks! Start your morning off right and fuel your body with the supplements it needs. Need more breakfast thoughts?

Lunch: Homestyle Mac and Cheese

A delectable lunch (or supper) formula that will be enjoyed by all! All things considered, how would you disapprove of a messy encouraging dish this way!

F-Factor puts a sound turn on a conventional formula by utilizing fixings like high-fiber pasta, Greek cream cheddar, without fat cheddar and a few other supplement rich and delightful fixings.

Tidbit: Peanut Butter Swirl

We as a whole get a sweet tooth wanting every once in a while however when that hankering strikes make certain to try these nutty spread twirl bars out!

This wanton formula utilizes fixings like chocolate protein powder, fine wheat grain, and powdered nutty spread to help keep these bars tasting scrumptious and brimming with nourishment. Try not to stress, these bars are still scrumptiously sweet (because of a F-Factor-affirmed sugar) and will make them return for additional.

Tidbit: Double Chocolate F-Factor Muffins

Biscuits make incredible in a hurry snacks so help yourself out and make a group of these flavorful chocolate F-Factor Muffins. Each serving contains 207 calories, 16 grams of fiber and 24 grams of protein.

Is the F-Factor Diet Healthy?

Since we've secured the fundamentals, here are the nourishment realities about the F-Factor Diet, directly from Harris-Pincus and Kris Sollid, R.D., ranking executive of sustenance interchanges for the International Food Information Council (IFIC) Foundation in Washington, D.C.

1. Fiber IS incredible for you.

Basically, Americans devour too many refined grains and high sugar nourishments that don't give satisfactory supplements and fiber, says Harris-Pincus.

"Nourishments that are high in fiber are solid, supplement thick nourishments like organic products, veggies, nuts, beans, seeds, and entire grains," she says. "You ought to eat these plant-based nourishments as most of your day by day consumption—notwithstanding lean proteins. They contain basic supplements, for example, nutrients, minerals, cancer prevention agents, and phytochemicals."

Those variables imply that "fiber assists with diminishing the danger of cardiovascular ailment by bringing down blood cholesterol, lessening circulatory strain, diminishing irritation," says Sollid. It's additionally been connected to bring down the danger of numerous diseases.

It likewise changes the rate at which your stomach related framework forms nourishments, making you more ordinary and boosting the strength of your gut microbiota, includes Sollid. (Related: Is the Microbiome Diet the Best Way to Promote Gut Health?)

"Fiber-rich nourishments additionally will in general give more volume than lower-fiber nourishments, which is thought to produce a more noteworthy sentiment of completion in less calories," she says. "Also, high-fiber nourishments will expect you to bite more. This basic move implies it makes longer to eat, which could likewise prompt eating less calories by and large." (Related: These Health Benefits of Fiber Make It the Most Important Nutrient In Your Diet)

2. In any case, know: you can devour an excessive amount of fiber.

All that being stated, "you can try too hard with fiber, so attempt to expand your fiber consumption bit by bit after some time and drink a lot of liquids at the same time," says Sollid. "An excessive amount of excessively fast, and not drinking abundant liquids during the F-Factor diet—or any high-fiber diet—can add to sickness or clogging." (Learn more about what can happen when you eat an excess of fiber.)

3. There's not only one sort of fiber.

In fact, "net carbs" don't have a legitimate definition, and the term isn't acknowledged by the Food and Drug Administration (FDA) or the American Diabetes Association, says Harris-Pincus.

Be that as it may, the distinction among solvent and insoluble fiber is characterized by the FDA:

"Solvent fiber disintegrates in water to shape a thick gel-like substance in the stomach. It is separated by microbes in the internal organ and gives a few calories."

"Insoluble fiber doesn't break up in water and goes through the gastrointestinal plot moderately flawless and, in this manner, isn't a wellspring of calories."

Since certain filaments are halfway edible and give two or three calories for every gram, Harris-Pincus suggests that people with Type 1 diabetes who are following the F-Factor diet (or any eating routine arrangement) ought to be directed by an enrolled dietitian or specialist. (Related: Can the Keto Diet Help with Type 2 Diabetes?)

4. You despite everything should be "calorie mindful" on the F-Factor diet.

You tally and track carbs and fiber on the F-Factor diet, yet it's as yet critical to be calorie mindful (no should be a calorie counter!), says Harris-Pincus. (Related: Counting Calories Helped Me Lose Weight—But Then I Developed an Eating Disorder)

"The more fiber you devour from supplement thick nourishments, the more fulfilled you are," she says.

In any case, you can without much of a stretch succumb to expending on a greater number of calories than you may might suspect.

"Frequently individuals accept that they are devouring 'solid' food, yet the segments are too enormous given then calorie substance, for example, avocados or nuts," says Harris-Pincus. "I generally suggest estimating those higher-fat and more fatty things when attempting to shed pounds on any eating routine."

Main concern: The F-Factor Diet might be advantageous for weight reduction in case you're searching for an eating regimen plan that doesn't require tallying calories. All things considered, fiber can help you subtly top off.

"Eventually, the quantity of calories you expend will decide how your weight changes," says Sollid. "In any case, fiber can assume a job in that. Some high-fiber nourishments are additionally low in calories, similar to vegetables, and eating an assortment of fiber-rich nourishments can help keep you feeling fulfilled by conveying a bigger volume of food to help keep you feeling full with less calories."

Simply remember to include another significant "F" to this intend to keep your muscles solid and your heart sound: wellness.

What Is the F-Factor Diet? Why

The "F" in F-Factor diet doesn't represent trend. Enlisted dietitian Tanya Zuckerbrot's book The F-Factor Diet: Discover the Secret to Permanent Weight Loss, first turned out in 2006, and her fiber-powered way to deal with good dieting has now stayed for longer than 10 years. Numerous celebs (like Katie Couric) have attempted the arrangement, and dissimilar to other popular "detoxes", this technique really has strong science behind it that could assist you with getting thinner — for good

"What I love about F-Factor is that it makes an arrangement wherein eating genuine, healthy nourishments and organizing supplement thick dinners and tidbits is straightforward and versatile to your own needs and propensities — without dispensing with anything or requiring some kind of extraordinary limitation," says Jaclyn London, MS, RD, CDN, Nutrition Director at the Good Housekeeping Institute.

This is what else you should think about the F-Factor Diet.

What is the F-Factor diet?

The F-Factor diet centers around getting enough fiber in your eating routine. What's so otherworldly about fiber? "It's a non-absorbable starch that is found on the planet's ideal, most nutritious nourishments — veggies, natural product, vegetables, nuts, seeds, and 100% entire grains," London says.

Following quite a while of working with customers with diabetes and coronary illness, Zuckerbrot understood that eating more fiber helped individuals not just oversee glucose levels and lower cholesterol, yet additionally get in shape. Other than showing up in a large number of bravo nourishments, fiber additionally tops you off so you're not feeling denied.

"These patients were just inclination more full for the duration of the day on less calories, which prompted weight reduction without hunger," Zuckerbrot said in a meeting with Camille Styles.

The arrangement endorses eating three fiber-filled dinners and a nibble every day, stacking up on sound carbs and lean protein, yet additionally getting a charge out of suppers out and the incidental beverage. So as to keep up long haul achievement, shouldn't limit and deny — consequently the "perpetual" some portion of the title. You can get all the points of interest in the book, yet the arrangement incorporates three general stages:

Kicking off Weight Loss: Eat 35 grams of fiber and under 35 grams of net carbs (3 servings) every day.

Proceeded with Weight Loss: Aim for in any event 35 grams of fiber and under 75 grams of net carbs (6 servings) every day.

Upkeep Eating: Aim for in any event 35 grams of fiber and under 125 grams of net carbs (9 servings) every day.

What number of grams of fiber would it be advisable for me to eat on the F-Factor Diet?

At each phase of the F-Factor diet, you should plan to eat in any event 35 grams of fiber for every day. That is not a discretionary number. The Dietary Guidelines for Americans suggests grown-ups expend between 28-35 grams of fiber day by day relying upon your age and sexual orientation. Nonetheless, just a simple 5% of us of draw near to that objective, as indicated by a recent report distributed in the American Journal of Lifestyle Medicine.

What do you eat on the F-Factor Diet?

No food is authoritatively beyond reach on the F-Factor diet. Rather, it's everything about including more fiber-full vegetables, organic products, beans, and entire grains to your plate.

All things considered, the main period of the eating regimen requests that you stay away from starches and dull vegetables, most dairy, and greasy meats. In any case, this part goes on for just fourteen days. From that point onward, you can proceed onward to Phase 2 and Phase 3, which place no limitations on any nourishments — yet you do need to hit that 35 grams of fiber benchmark.

Do as such by stacking up on these fiber-full nourishments, as recorded by the Dietary Guidelines for Americans:

Heartbeats: beans, peas, chickpeas, lentils

Entire Grains: bulgur, quinoa, grain, entire grain bread, high-fiber oat, destroyed wheat oat, wheat oat, rye saltines, entire wheat pasta, air-popped popcorn

Organic products: apples, pears, raspberries, blackberries, figs, oranges, bananas, guava, dates

Vegetables: artichokes, avocado, collards, yam, pumpkin, parsnips, squash

Nuts and Seeds: pumpkin seeds, chia seeds, sunflower seeds, almonds, pistachios, walnuts, hazelnuts, peanuts

"Regardless of whether you're picking in on F-Factor or not, pick nourishments that are in their most healthy state as could reasonably be expected, inside the bounds of your financial plan and sense of taste," London prompts. "Oranges versus squeezed orange, broiled veggies versus veggie chips, etc."

Does the F-Factor Diet truly work?

Truly, the F-Factor diet can assist you with getting in shape if that is your objective. "Fiber, explicitly, is fundamental to progress on the F-Factor diet, as it permits you to eat the starches vital for vitality without putting on weight," Zuckerbrot revealed to Camille Styles. "At the point when you follow an eating regimen wealthy in fiber you feel full subsequent to eating – so you'll for the most part eat less for the duration of the day."

The arrangement can likewise profit you in different manners. "While it'll work for weight reduction, the inhabitants of the arrangement make it maintainable for anybody to settle on more advantageous decisions in light of the fact that the program makes them organize genuine, entire nourishments that are supplement thick — without being a finished nap," London says.

She cherishes that it advances eating more heartbeats, veggies, entire grains, and organic product, yet alerts that encircling everything as far as "fiber" could let you dismiss eating and getting a charge out of genuine food.

"Organize healthy, feeding nourishments before reconsidering all that you eat as far as the supplements it contains," London exhorts. "We profit by sustenance from various sources and encounters — getting a charge out of food ought to be up front, not simply concentrating on one single supplement!"

Counting calories can be troublesome, particularly on the off chance that you've chosen to do everything all alone. Be that as it may, a little accommodating exhortation, a couple of plans, and two or three examples of overcoming adversity can go far. That is the reason we chose to talk with F-Factor author Tanya Zuckerbrot, MS, RD, about how to make counting calories feasible. Not at all like other get-healthy plans, the F-Factor diet allows you to feast out, drink your preferred grown-up refreshments, and work out less while as yet getting thinner.

What does the F-Factor diet plan incorporate?

While different eating regimens power weight watchers to take out fats and carbs, the F-Factor diet is tied in with including fiber.

"Most eating regimens depend on exclusion — to accomplish weight reduction, certain nourishments like starches or fats, or lifestyles, such as feasting out or drinking, are excluded," Zuckerbrot said. "The issue with this is it leaves calorie counters feeling ravenous, denied, and disappointed. The F-Factor Program, then again, depends on option — you add fiber into your eating regimen to get more fit, so there are no sentiments of hardship and forswearing, which frequently keeps weight watchers down, eventually making them come up short."

As such, rather than starving, health food nuts will at last get the opportunity to feel full — yet the weight will at present fall off. This, Zuckerbrot accepts, is the way to remaining persuaded. So how does the F-Factor diet chip away at an ordinary premise?

"F-Factor is intended to fit consistently into people groups' lives so they can stay on track. From the very first moment on F-Factor, you can feast out and drink liquor, invest less energy at the rec center, eat starches and normal suppers (breakfast, lunch, bite, supper, and treat), and still get more fit. These standards are outlandish to what we accept about weight reduction, genuinely making it a freeing plan," Zuckerbrot proceeded. "Finally, F-Factor is about training. It shows individuals how to eat forever, and how to keep up their weight reduction (which amends the principal issue of prevailing fashion eats less carbs). This last factor just adds to what in particular makes F-Factor such an economical arrangement."

What to Eat on F-Factor Diet

Members on the F-Factor diet ought to eat four suppers every day: breakfast, lunch, a bite, and supper.

"The blend of fiber and protein keeps you feeling full for the longest timeframe on the least calories," Zuckerbrot said. "The more full you feel after a supper, the more uncertain you'll be to indulge at the following feast and in this way, the more probable you'll be to get in shape."

F-Factor Diet Sample Menu

What might an example day of eating F-Factor diet nourishments involve? Shockingly, it's not very unique in relation to what you're as of now eating. This is what a run of the mill day on a F-

Factor feast plan would resemble, as per Zuckerbrot:

Breakfast: Nonfat plain Greek yogurt with 1/2 cup of high-fiber oat and 1 cup of berries

Lunch: Miso soup, naruto move, 2 hand rolls (no rice), and serving of mixed greens with ginger dressing

Tidbit: F-Factor Pizzas (4 high-fiber wafers finished off with low-fat curds or mozzarella cheddar, pureed tomatoes, and a sprinkle of parmesan cheddar, microwaved until dissolved.) Tip — By eating a nibble two hours before supper, you won't go into supper eager and can settle on more advantageous choices.

Supper: Steamed entire artichoke, filet mignon (3 oz. for ladies, 6 oz. for men), steamed asparagus and a merited glass (or two) of wine or spirits on the rocks

Wine and pizza? The F-Factor diet nourishments are ones we could get behind! In any case, pause, it shows signs of improvement: There are additionally hotcakes and waffles included.

The most effective method to Eat More F-Factor Diet Foods

In case you're uncertain of how to fuse fiber into your eating routine, the F-Factor site has an assortment of plans to move you, from Creamy Baked Spinach and Artichoke Dip to Baked Spaghetti Pie. Yum! Tired of being on the web? Look at the book The F-Factor Diet ($11, Amazon), which you can convey with you any place you go.

"I love our high-fiber flapjack and Step 1 Waffle plans — made with only a couple of straightforward fixings, this hotcake packs in 19 grams of protein and 16 grams of fiber for under 225 calories, and it very well may be made into something flavorful or sweet," Zuckerbrot said. "It's immediately become a staple formula for my customers."

F-Factor Diet Results

What would dieters be able to hope to pick up from keeping the F-Factor diet rules? Something other than weight reduction, that is without a doubt. Expanded vitality, a compliment stomach, more clear skin, improved rest, improved cholesterol levels, and better-oversaw glucose levels are only a couple of the advantages of the F-Factor diet, as per Zuckerbrot.

"At last, diet bests practice with regards to weight reduction," Zuckerbrot said. "I tell customers, let F-Factor be your cardio. Individuals do cardio to make a caloric shortfall, yet cardio can invigorate hunger and hinder weight reduction endeavors. Rather, make a caloric shortfall by eating an eating routine high in fiber, similar to F-Factor. The explanation this works is on the grounds that eating fiber consumes calories — fiber can't be processed, so it fires up digestion. The more fiber you're eating, the more calories your body consumes very still. I don't think about you, yet I'd preferably eat fiber over invest more energy in the treadmill."

Sounds like Zuckerbrot gets us totally! No big surprise celebs acclaim the F-Factor diet — and why such a significant number of individuals can stay with it long haul. What do you believe, is it worth a shot?

Everything necessary for an eating regimen to explode is a couple of famous people to begin humming about it. That is actually what occurred with the F-Factor diet after Megyn Kelly, Katie Couric, and Olivia Culpo raved about it. The eating regimen initially began getting buzz in 2006 after dietitian and F-Factor originator Tanya Zuckerbrot distributed the book, The F-Factor Diet: Discover the Secret to Permanent Weight Loss.

From that point forward, a lot of individuals have hopped onto the F-Factor train. Perhaps you've known about it, possibly you haven't. In case you're at all fluffy on the subtleties, we have answers to your inquiries: What's this about once more? What's more, how does the entire thing really work?

What is the F-Factor diet?

The eating regimen depends on four rules that sound really extraordinary: Eat carbs, eat out, drink liquor, turn out to be less. Obviously, it's somewhat more nuanced than that. The eating routine explicitly centers around consolidating lean proteins with high-fiber starches that are low in calories and keep you feeling full.

The eating regimen was established by enlisted dietitian Tanya Zuckerbrot, who has been in private practice in NYC for over 20 years.

How can it work?

The "F" in F-Factor means "fiber," and the eating routine is enthusiastic about that. It suggests that ladies have in any event 35 grams of fiber daily and that men have at least 38 grams of the stuff every day.

Fiber is a non-edible starch, and "one of the most significant dietary segments related with great wellbeing," says Sonya Angelone, RD, a representative for the Academy of Nutrition and Dietetics. "For more than 40 years, research contemplates have reliably demonstrated that dietary fiber is related with more beneficial cholesterol and glucose levels, is related with less obstruction and better gut work, less colon malignant growth, and assists with weight the board," Angelone says.

Fiber additionally helps top you off and remain fulfilled, so eating a lot of it can help lessen cravings for food numerous individuals experience on different weight control plans, says New York-based enrolled dietitian Jessica Cording.

Suppers incorporate things like chicken cacciatore, zucchini parmesan waffles, and rich mushroom asparagus risotto.

Is it solid?

It unquestionably can possibly be solid on the off chance that you approach it right. "This eating regimen is doubtlessly solid if entire insignificantly handled nourishments are picked," she says. "The advantage originates from eating entire nourishments." Cording concurs. Since the eating regimen isn't prohibitive, it makes it almost certain that individuals will stay with it. "Numerous individuals think that its engaging that they can in any case appreciate starches and liquor," she says.

For what reason would it be able to assist me with getting in shape?

"Since this eating regimen joins lean proteins with fiber—two supplements that assist you with remaining full—eating thusly can help fight off those sentiments of yearning that will in general wet blanket up when somebody is on a weight reduction diet," Cording says. What's more, on a psychological level, after an eating routine that stresses including more fiber as opposed to confining what you eat "can help abstain from worshiping prohibited nourishments that prompts obsession with those nourishments," she says.

High fiber nourishments likewise will in general be truly solid, and topping off on sound nourishments can prompt weight reduction. "High fiber nourishments are typically vegetables, natural products, entire grains, and vegetables," Angelone calls attention to. "Nourishments with fiber are plants (since fiber gives plants structure) and have less calories per volume that fats and proteins."

What would i be able to eat?

There are a couple of various ways you can move toward the eating routine. A lot of individuals purchase Zuckerbrot's book and take it from that point. There are heaps of plans on the F-Factor Diet's site that you can use for motivation, and Pinterest is pressed with them, as well.

Zuckerbrot likewise sells things on her site like F-Factor protein powder and protein bars, on the off chance that you need to kick things up a score. Furthermore, in case you're willing to dish out somewhat more cash, you can make a meeting with Zuckerbrot or one of her kindred F-Factor dietitians to get one-on-one training.

Do dietitians have any worries about this?

Since the F-Factor diet is a high fiber diet, Cording just suggests venturing up your fiber admission bit by bit "to maintain a strategic distance from stomach related uneasiness like gas, swelling, and stomach inconvenience." It's likewise a smart thought to drink bunches of water to keep things traveling through your GI plot, she says.

The eating regimen likewise doesn't address bit and hunger control. "A few people are overweight since they eat in any event, when full," Angelone says. "They might not have hunger hormones that manage craving appropriately, they may eat carelessly, and they may eat for passionate reasons. Simply eating more fiber, which fills the stomach more, may not be the solution for everybody's weight issues

Made in the USA
Middletown, DE
20 October 2023

41117792R00056